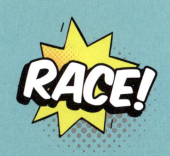
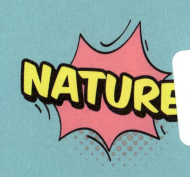

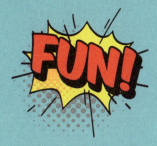
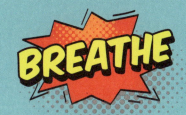
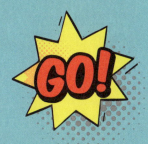
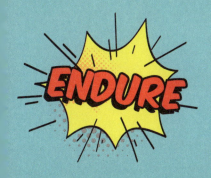
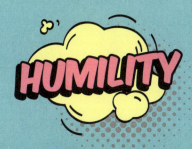
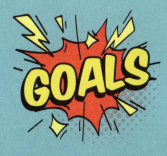
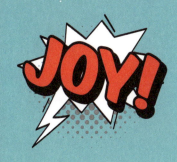
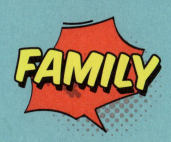
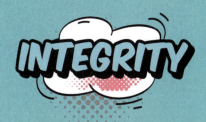

FOR MAX AND TURNER.
MAY YOU RUN WITH PURPOSE AND JOY.

FOR HAYLEY.
MAY YOU CHASE AND LEAD MAX AND TURNER WITH STRENGTH AND GRACE.

Text © 2019 Matt Sorenson
Illustrations © 2019 Andrew Langston
Designed by Dayle Hendrickson

All rights reserved. Published by G5 Active. G5 Active holds full and exclusive rights to My Mommy Runs and all related titles, logos, illustrations, and characters. No part of this book may be reproduced or transmitted in any form or by any means, electronic or mechanical, including photocopy, recording, or any storage and retrieval system now known or to be invented without written permission from G5 Active.

Printed in the United States

First Edition

ISBN: 978-1-7339146-0-4
Library of Congress Control Number: 2019903848

To order or contact the author, visit www.g5active.com
Follow @g5active on social media.

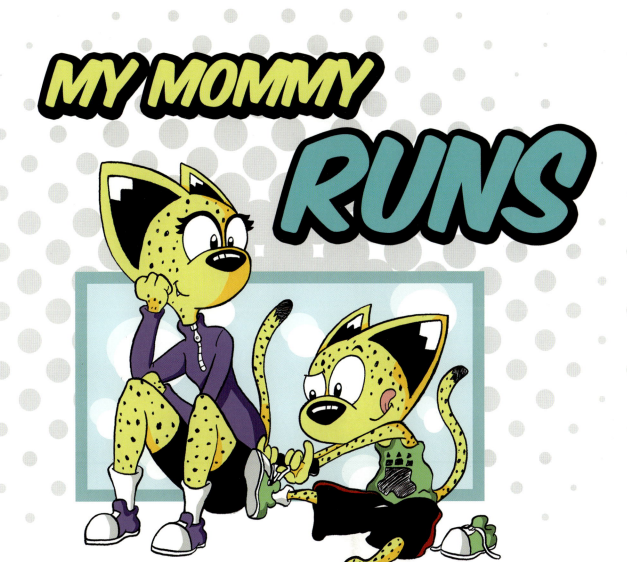

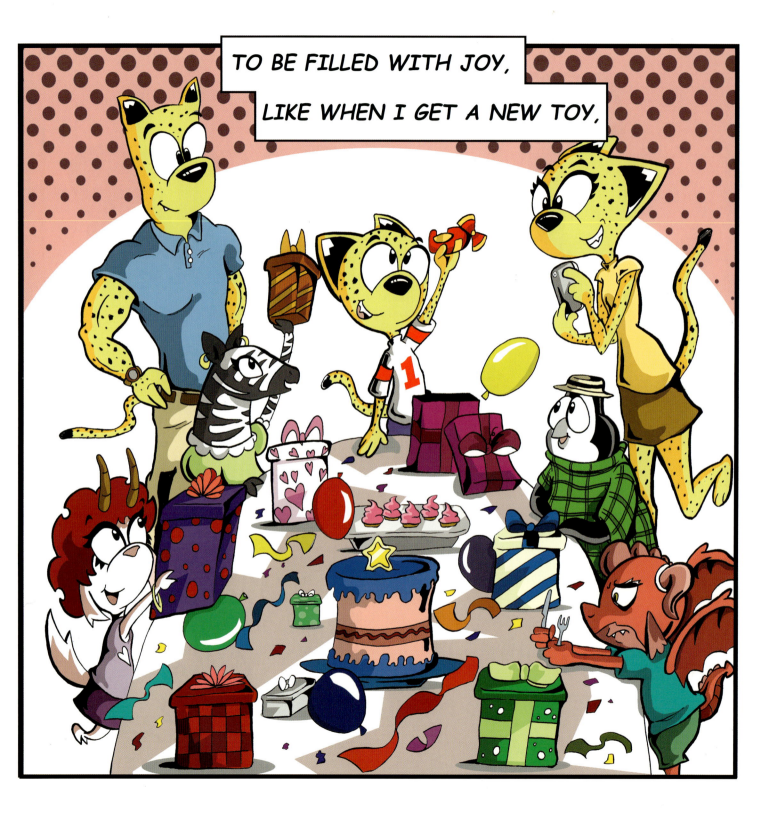

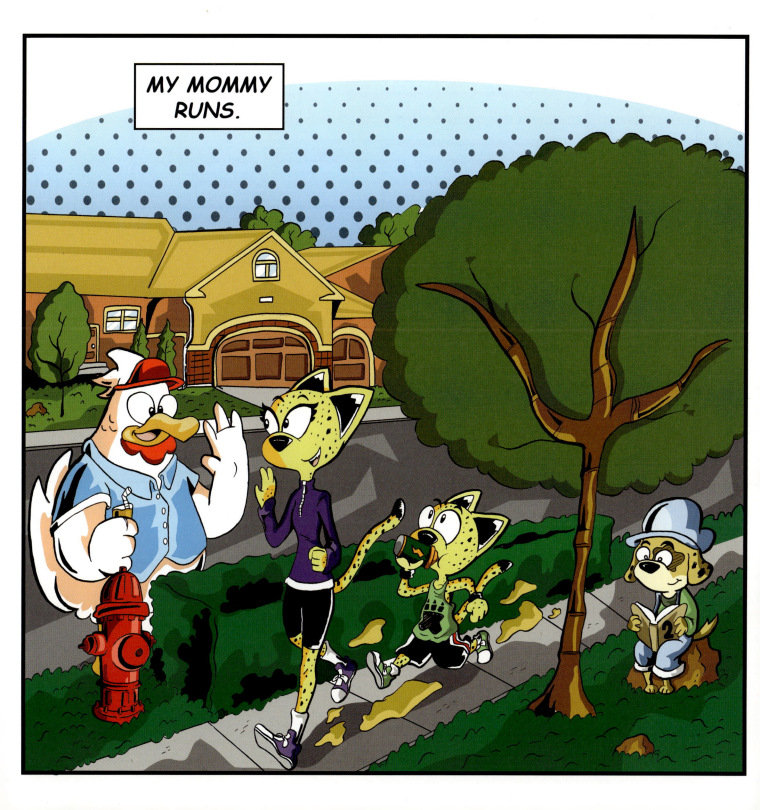

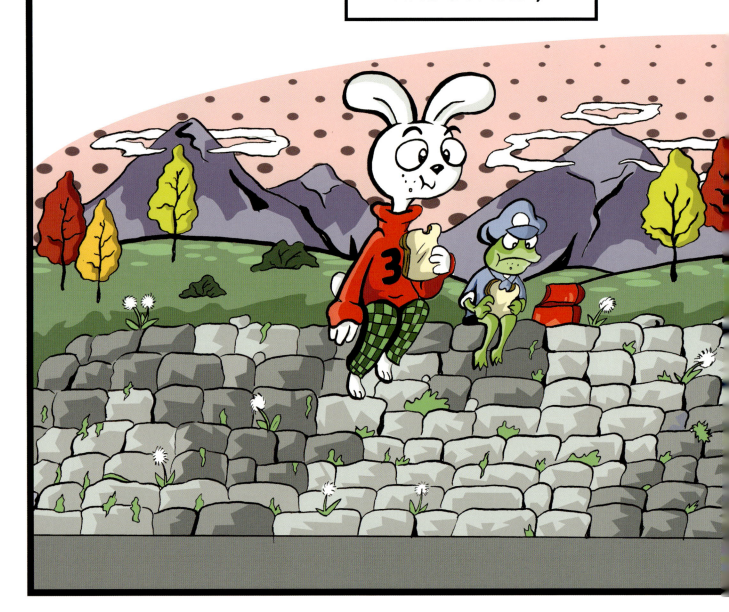

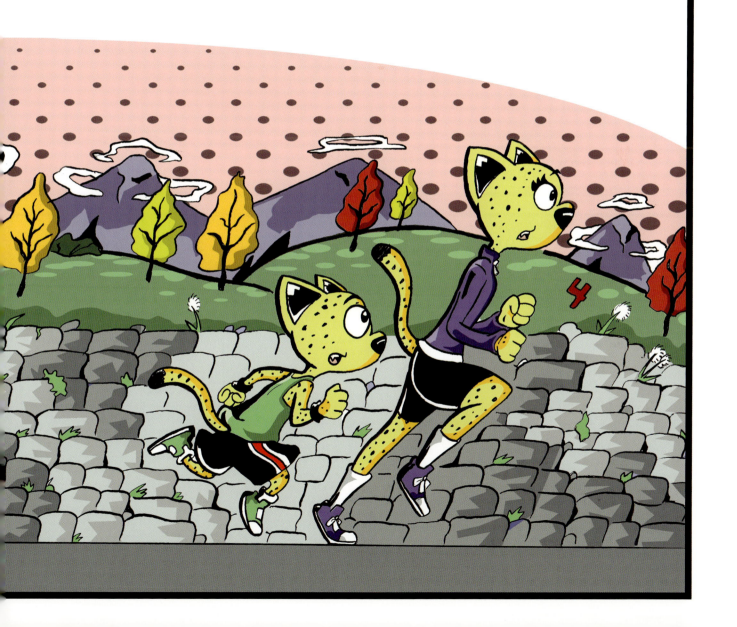
MY MOMMY RUNS.

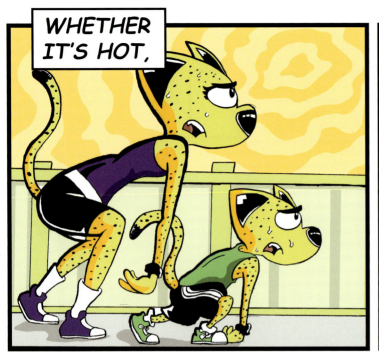
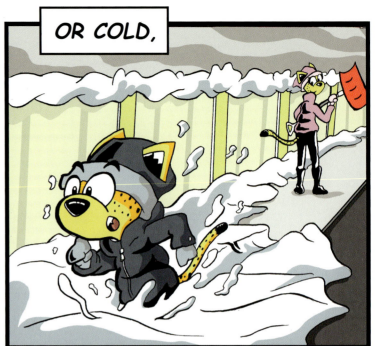
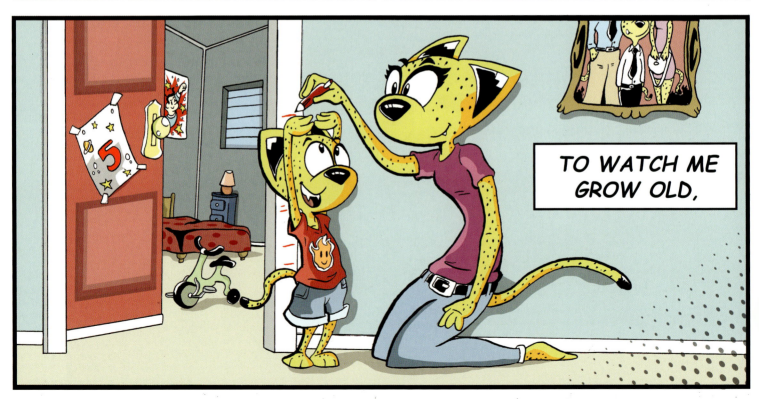

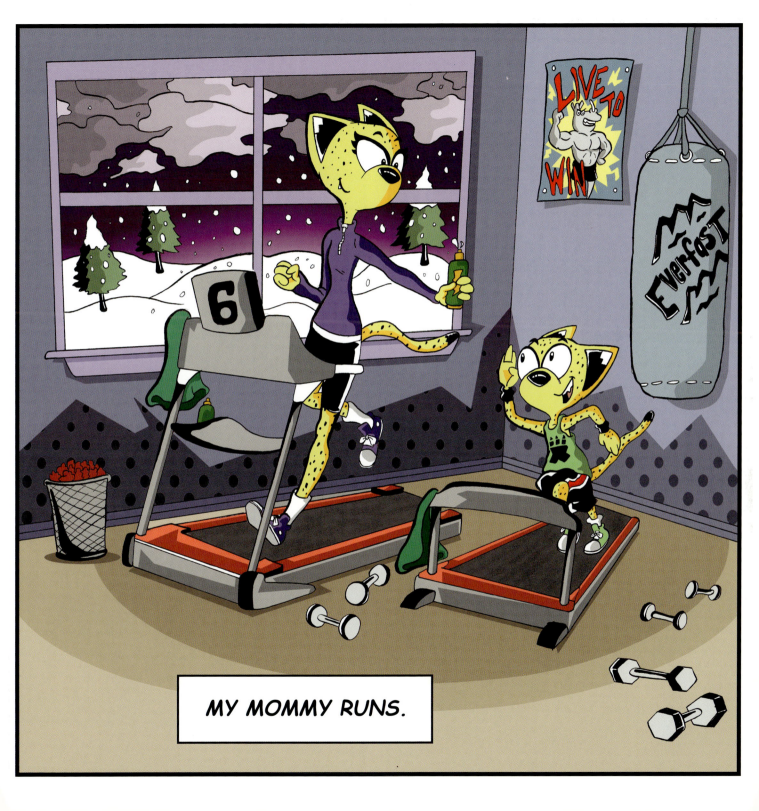

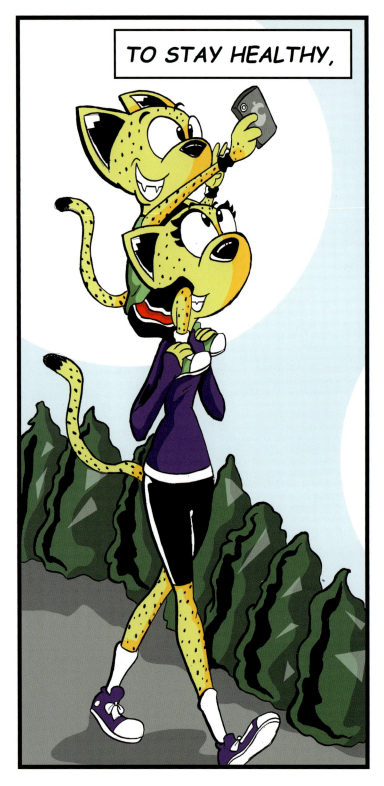
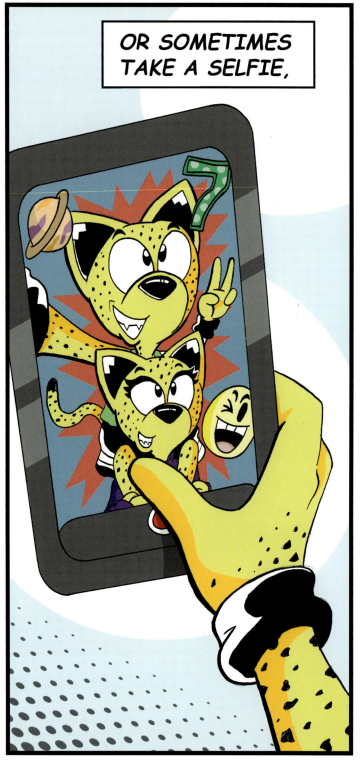

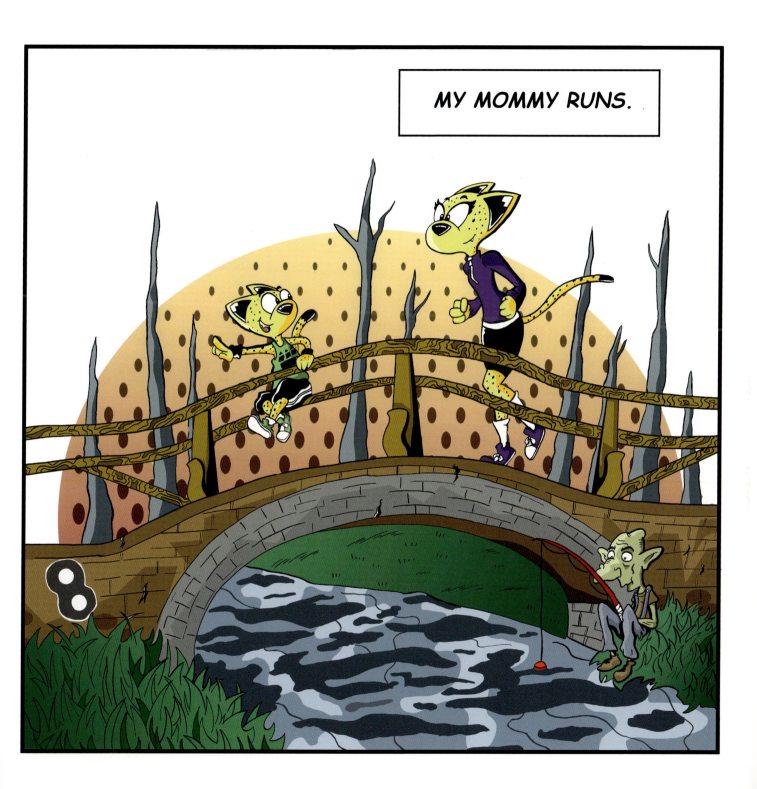

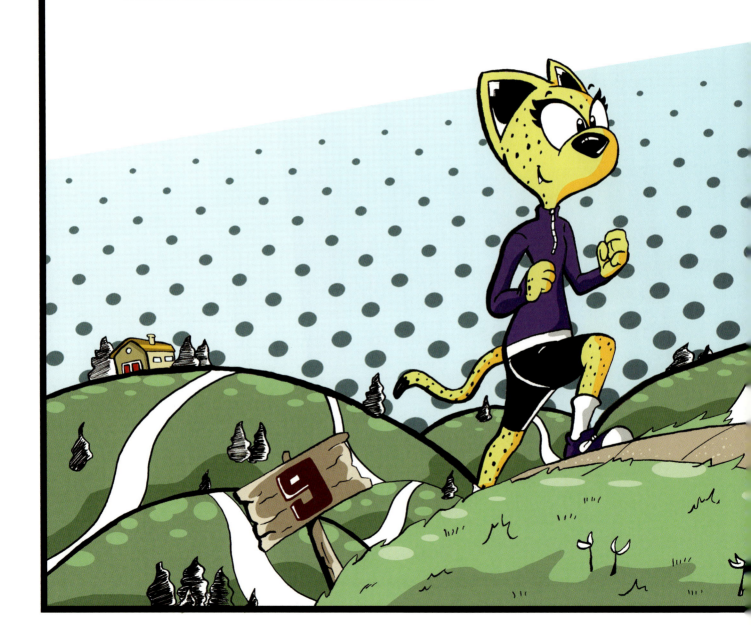

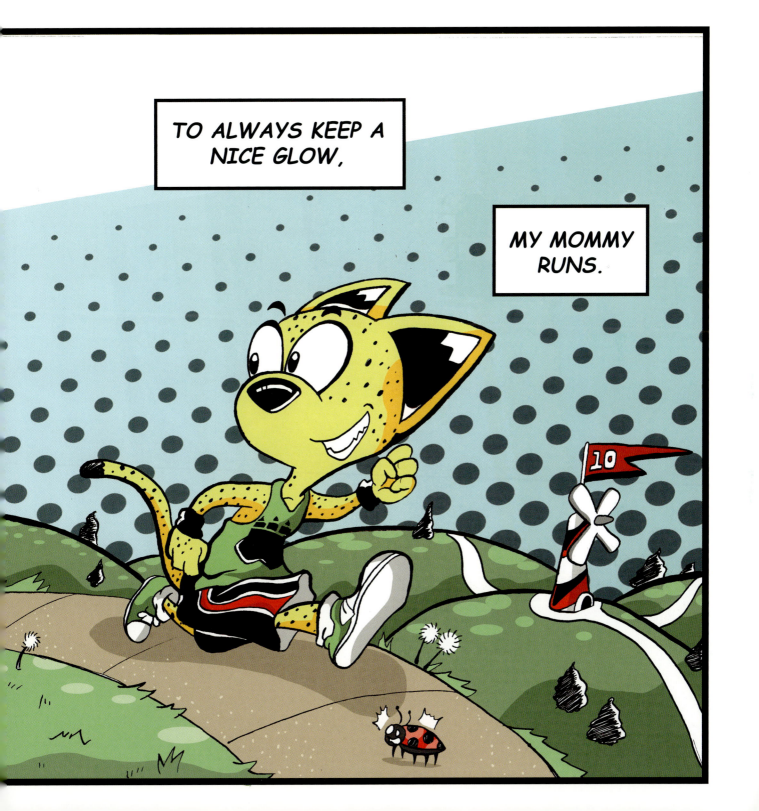

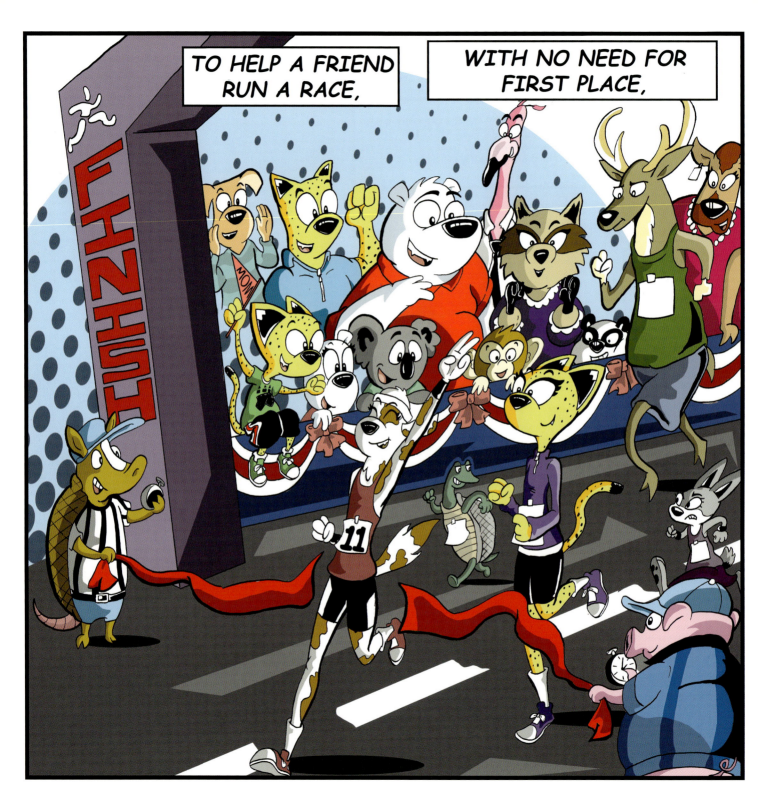

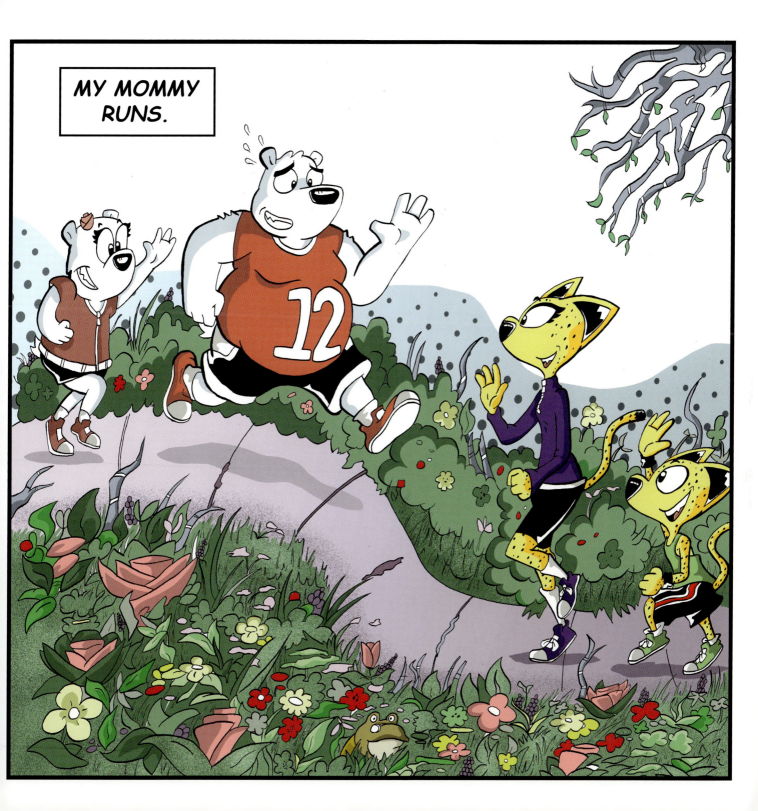

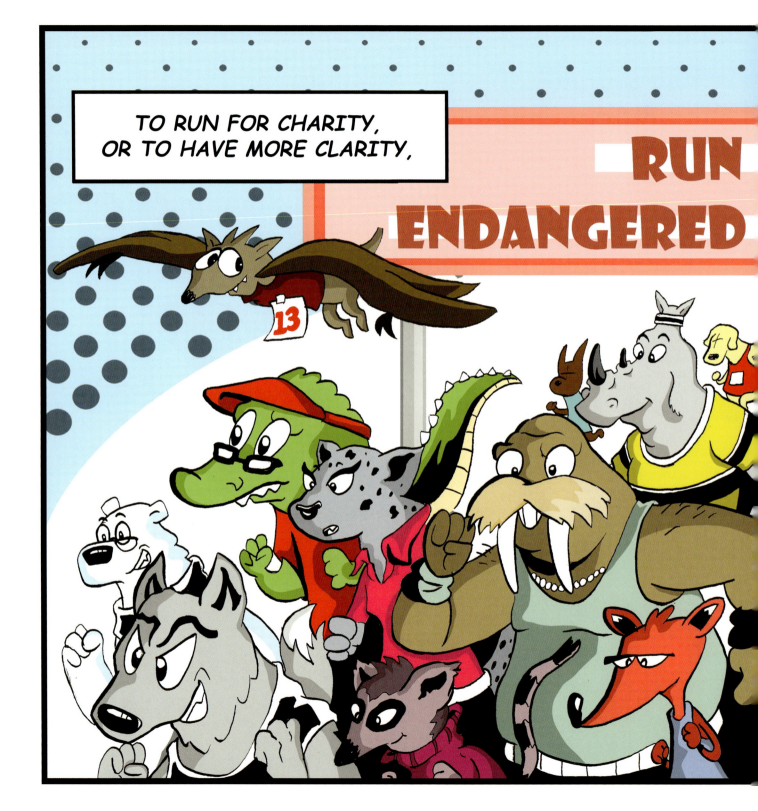

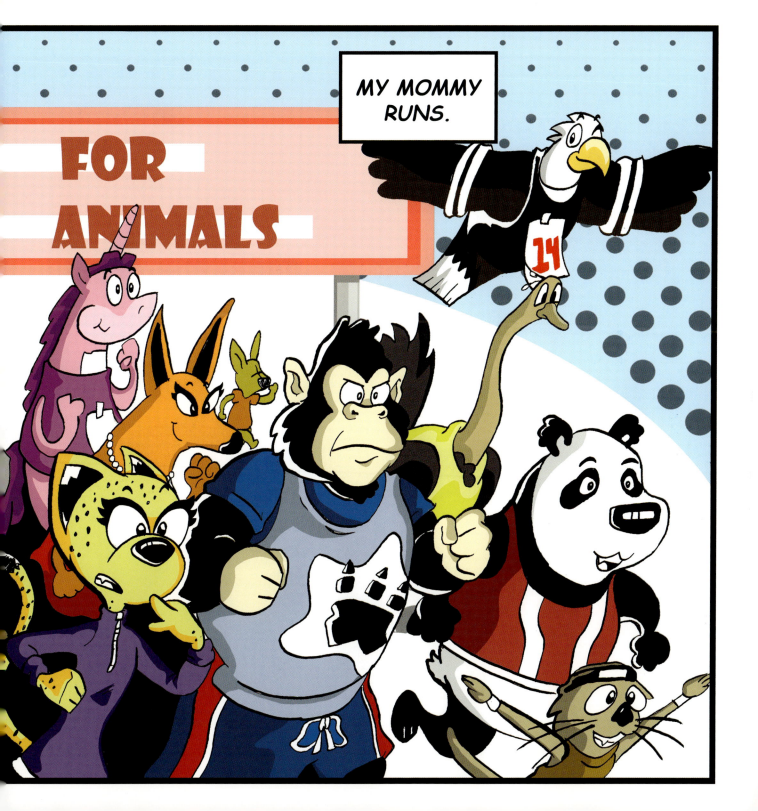

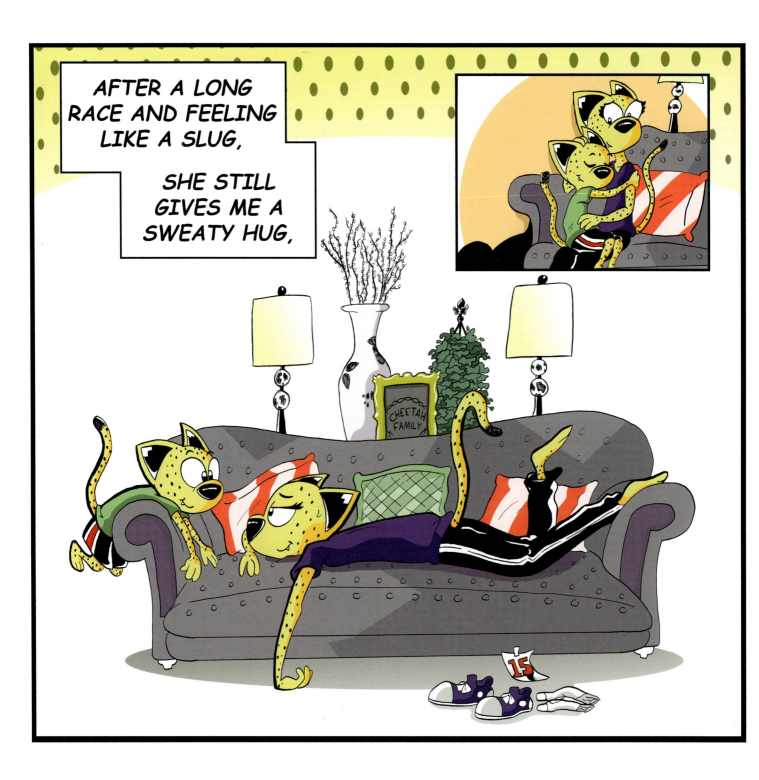

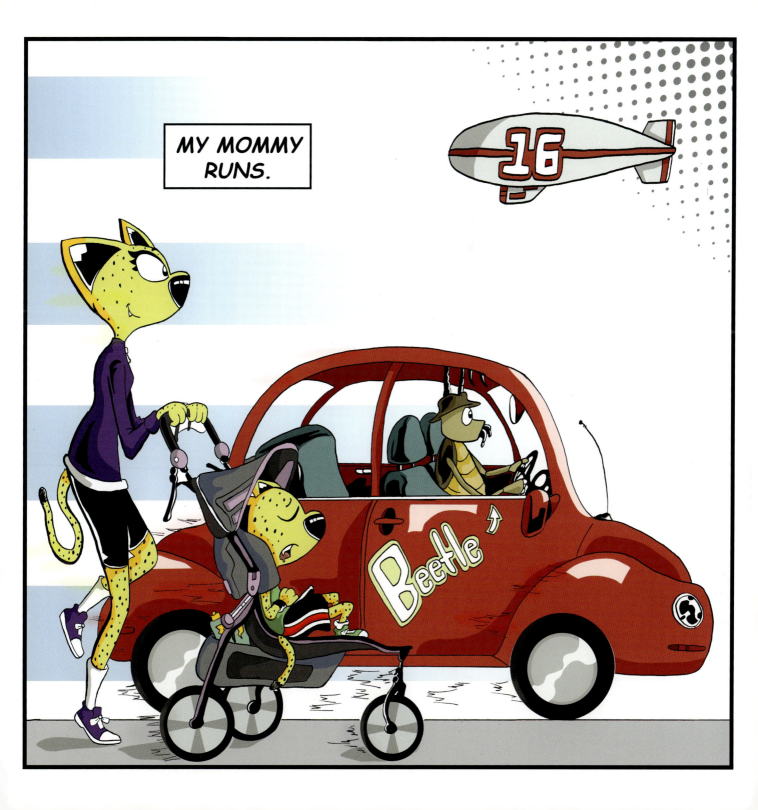

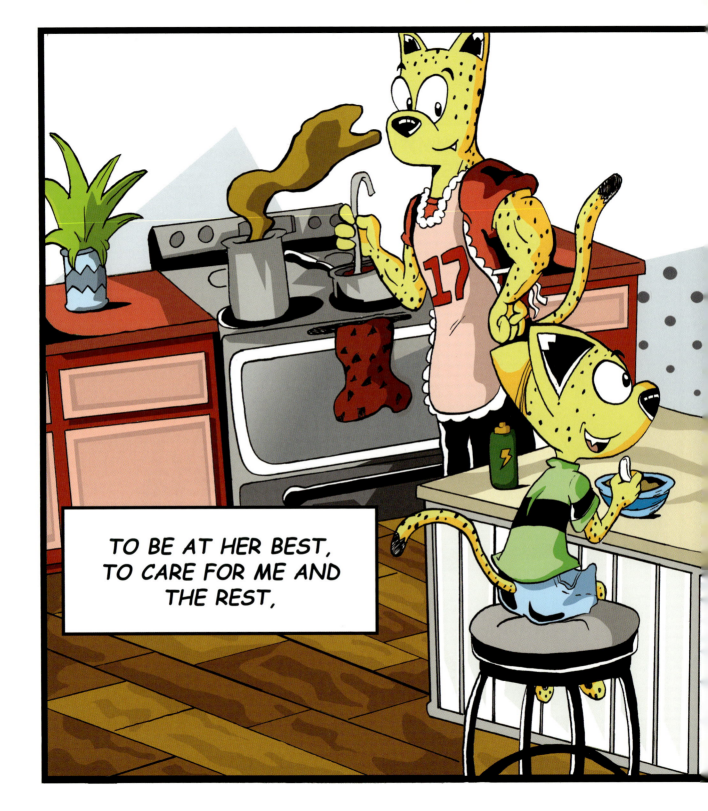

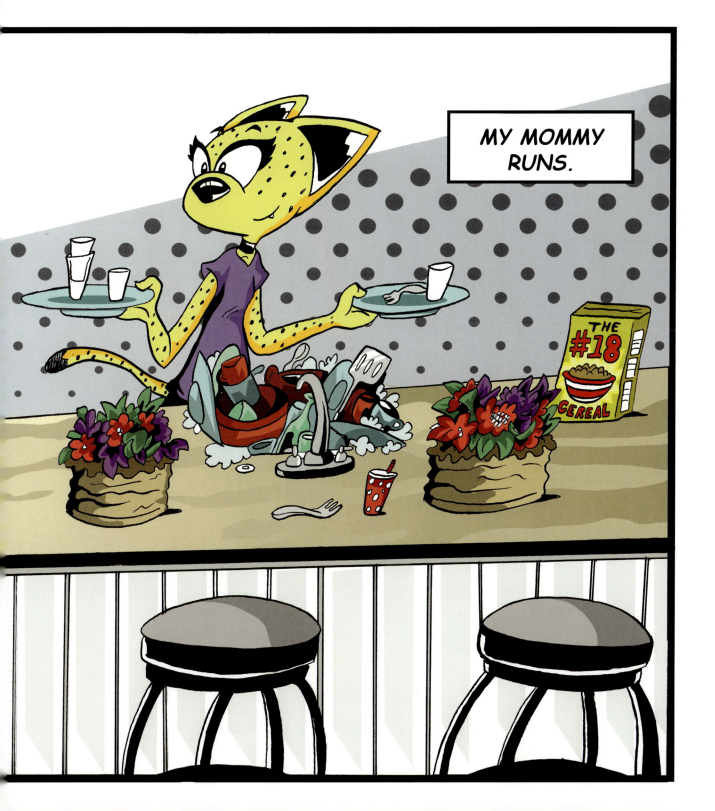

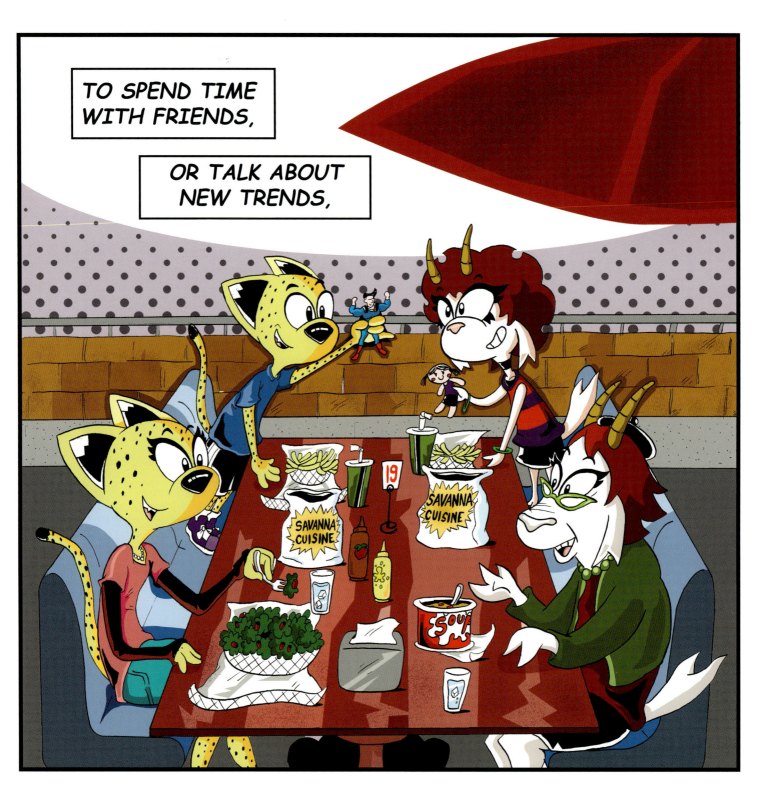

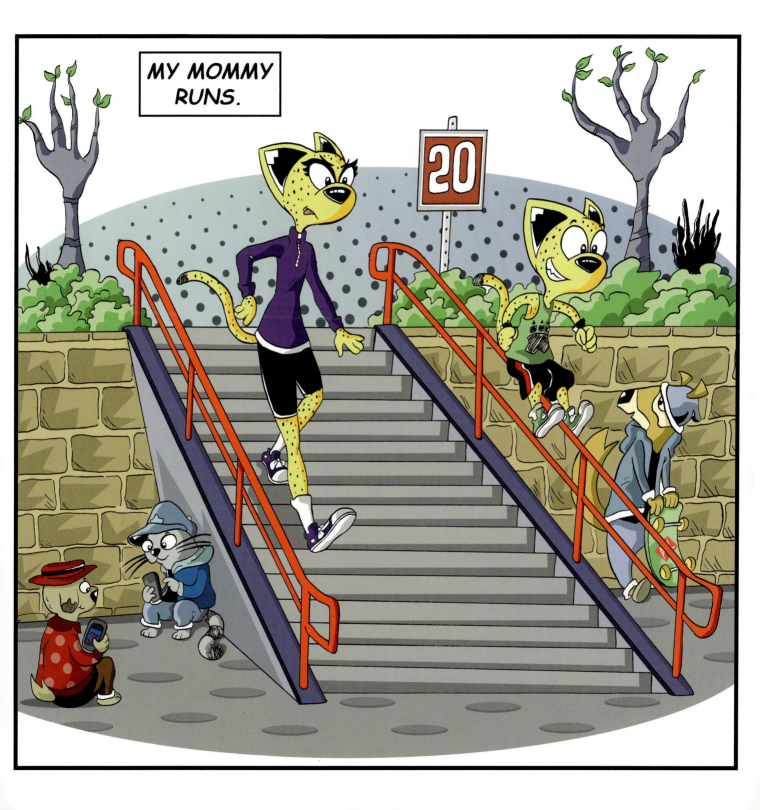

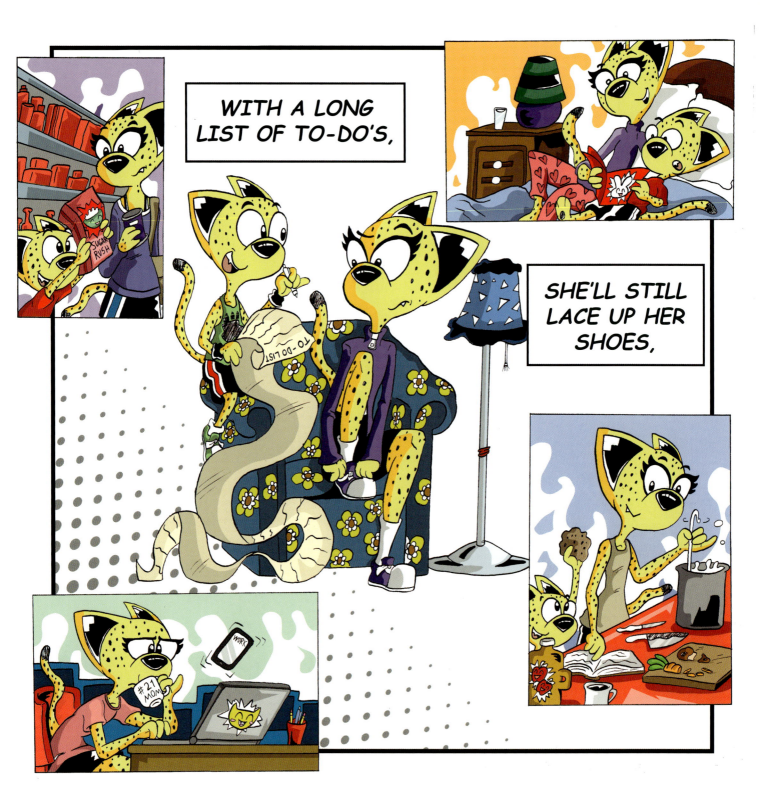

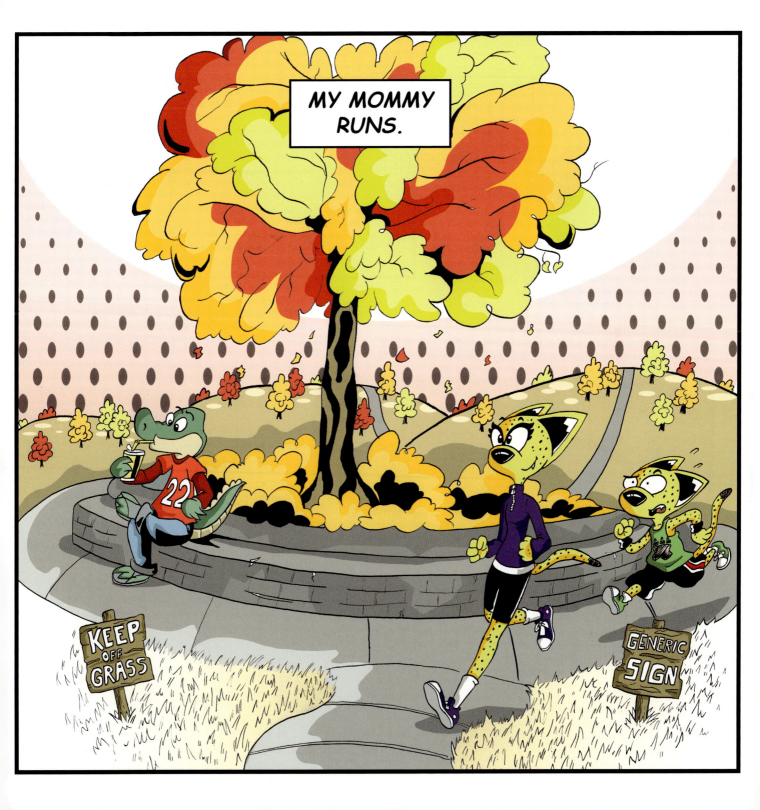

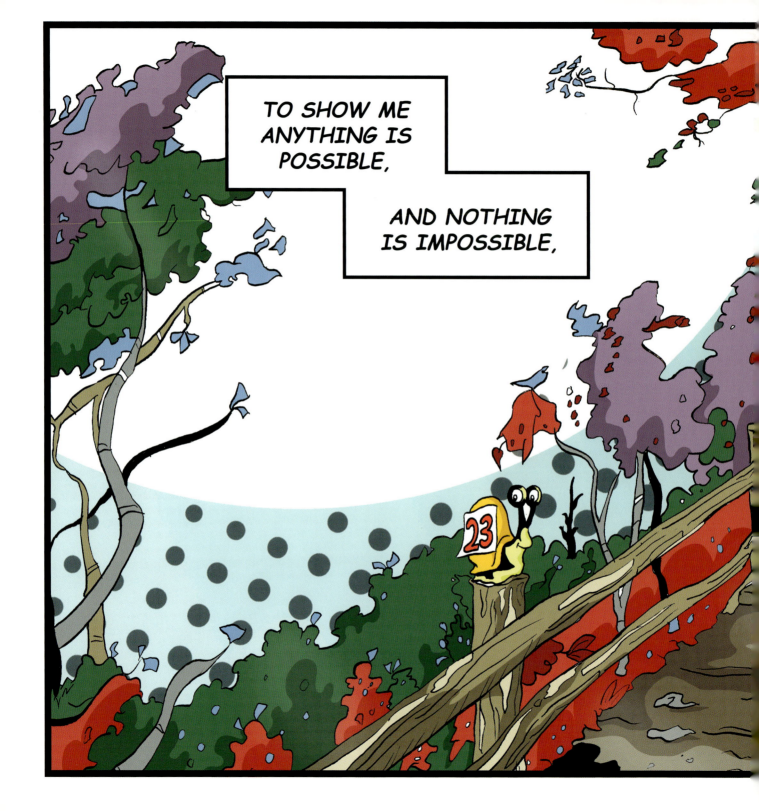

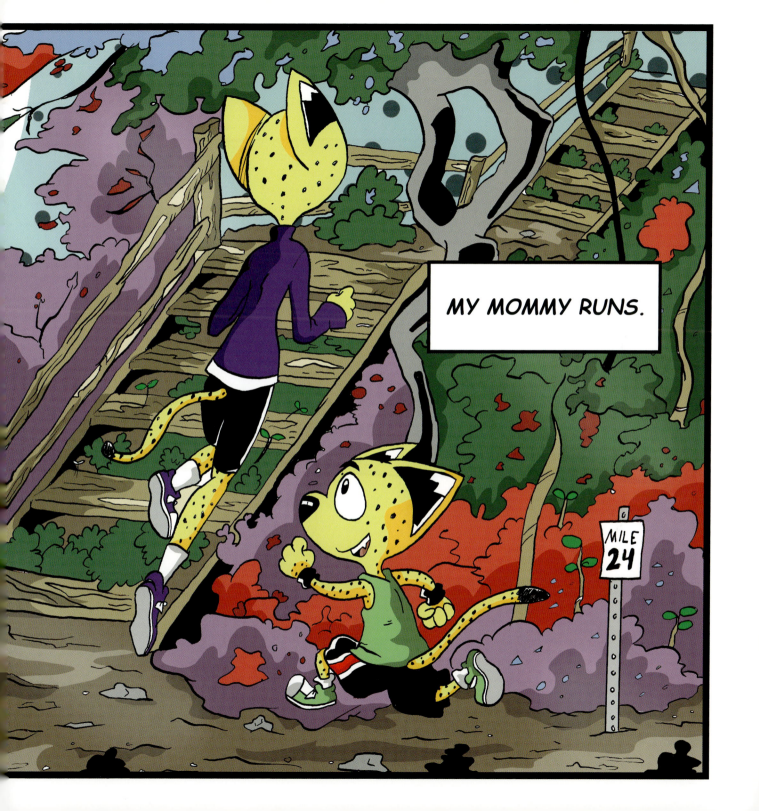

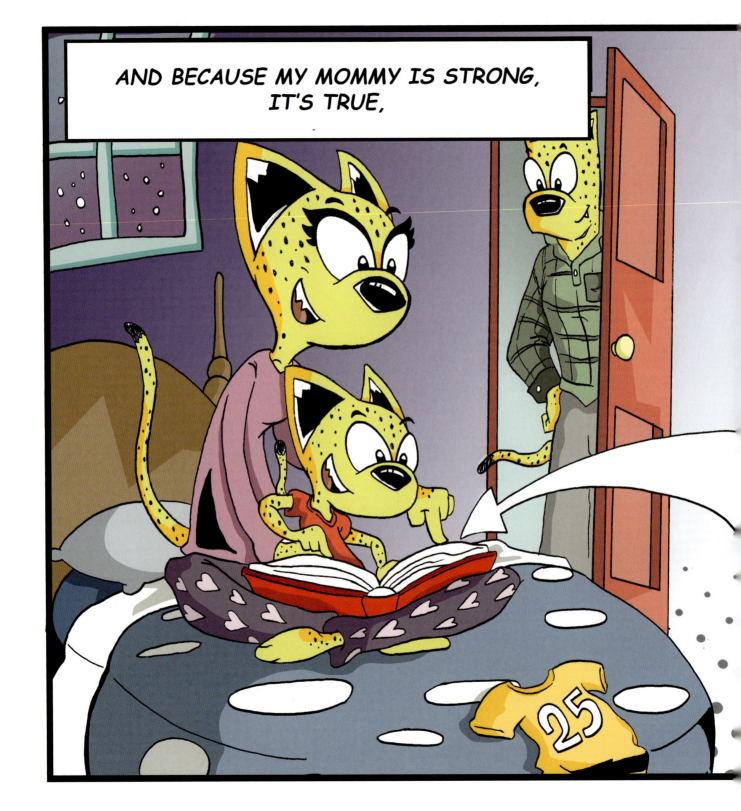

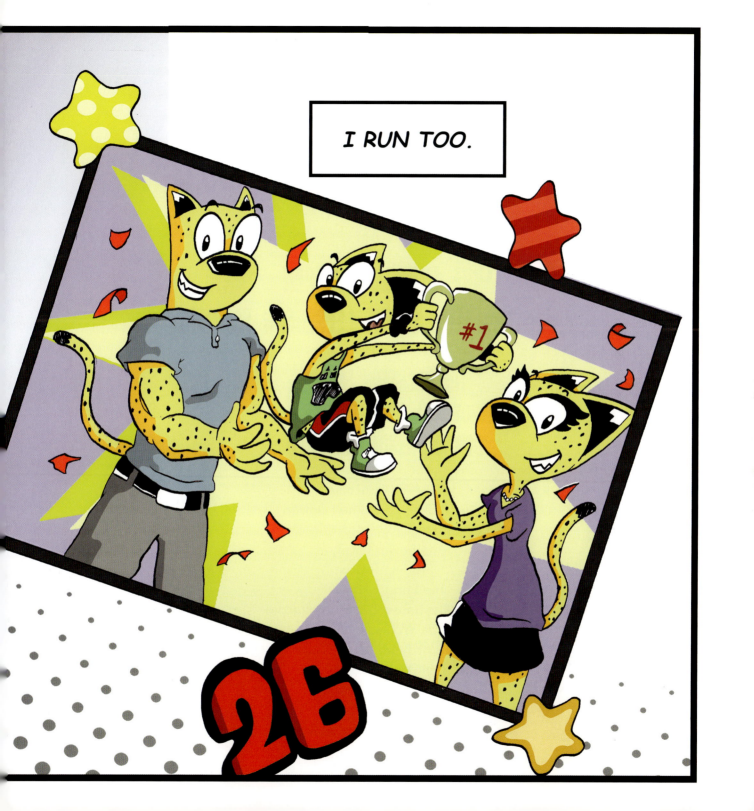

THANK YOU TO EVERYONE WHO MADE THIS BOOK A REALITY, ESPECIALLY:

MIKE AND JAN KAMPEN
GRANDMA WALTERS & THE LEESEBERG FAMILIES

THE BOCHATON FAMILY
TROY AND JENNY LANGSTON
DON AND LINDA SORENSON

Run4PRs Coaching
Knox, Blakely, and Rhett Dotson
Empower Family Chiropractic - Dr. J
The Brown Family
Starling Teams
The Enright Family
Ashley's Playhouse- Drop-in Childcare
The Wallin Family
Friends of Team World Vision
The Orozco Family
3100: Run and Become
The Telschow Family
Sheri Wall with A Matter of Rhyme

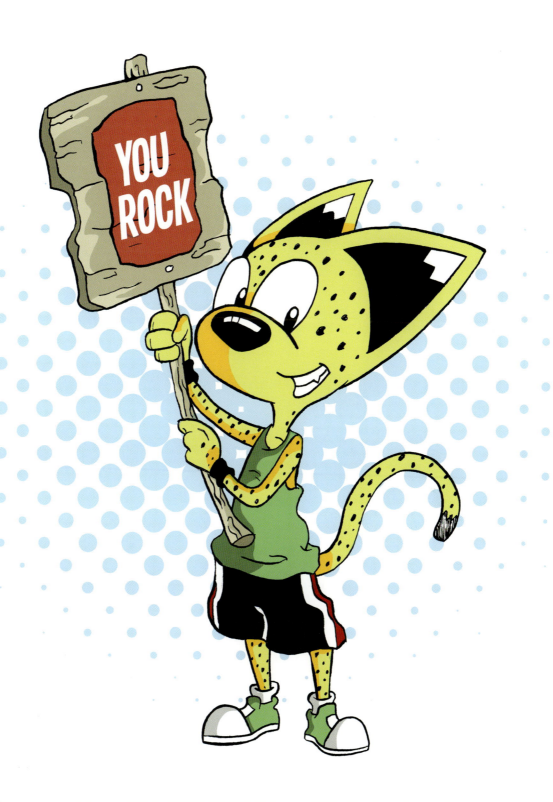

MY MOMMY RUNS BIBLE VERSES

IN LINE WITH G5 ACTIVE'S MISSION AND BELIEFS, HERE ARE SOME BIBLE VERSES SHOULD YOU CHOOSE TO EXPLORE THE THEMES OF SPECIFIC PAGES FURTHER.

Pages 1 & 2
ROMANS 15:13
PHILIPPIANS 4:4
PHILEMON 1:7

Pages 3 & 4
ISAIAH 40:31
GALATIANS 6:9
2 THESSALONIANS 3:13

Pages 5 & 6
JOHN 16:33
COLOSSIANS 1:11
JAMES 1:2-3

Pages 7 & 8
1 CORINTHIANS 6:19-20
1 TIMOTHY 4:8
3 JOHN 1:2

Pages 9 & 10
JEREMIAH 29:11
ROMANS 12:12
1 TIMOTHY 4:15

Pages 11 & 12
ECCLESIASTES 4:9-10
1 CORINTHIANS 10:24
PHILIPPIANS 2:3

Pages 13 & 14
PROVERBS 19:17
PHILIPPIANS 4:6-7
HEBREWS 13:16

Pages 15 & 16
ROMANS 5:3-4
1 CORINTHIANS 13:4-7
HEBREWS 12:11-12

Pages 17 & 18
PROVERBS 22:6
MATTHEW 11:28
HEBREWS 4:9-10

Pages 19 & 20
PROVERBS 27:17
PSALM 133:1
1 JOHN 4:21

Pages 21 & 22
PROVERBS 23:25
PROVERBS 31:17
PHILIPPIANS 2:14-15

Pages 23 & 24
MARK 10:27
LUKE 1:37
PHILIPPIANS 4:13

Pages 25 & 26
PSALM 73:26
PROVERBS 31:25
ISAIAH 40:29

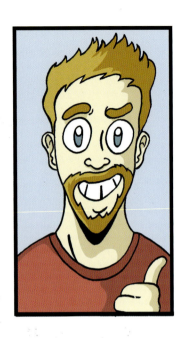

MATT SORENSON

How does a PhD in microbiology qualify a person to write a children's book? It doesn't. But what does, is a can-do, problem solving, collaborative, and lifelong learning personality. I hope all who read this book enjoy it and may you think about how you can use your ideas, talents, and time to make the world a better place.

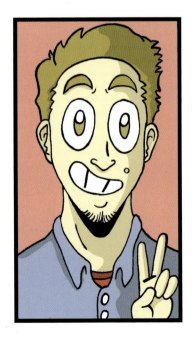

ANDREW LANGSTON

While I'm not a particularly talented artist I do pride myself on my cute animal characters. It is my sincerest wish that the readers of this book went "d'awwwww!" at least twice while looking through the pictures. Either that or children start doodling my characters on random scratch paper. I'd be happy either way.

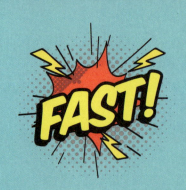 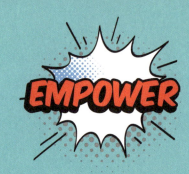 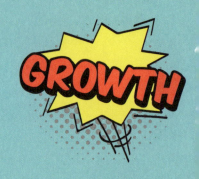
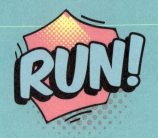 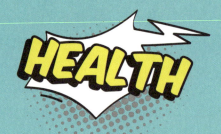 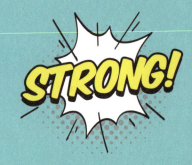
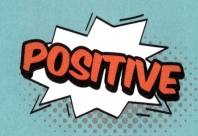 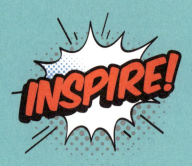 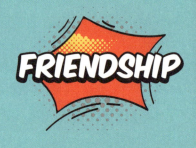
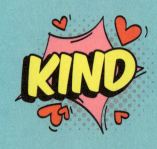 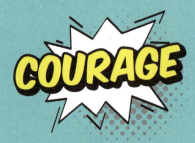 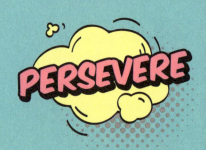